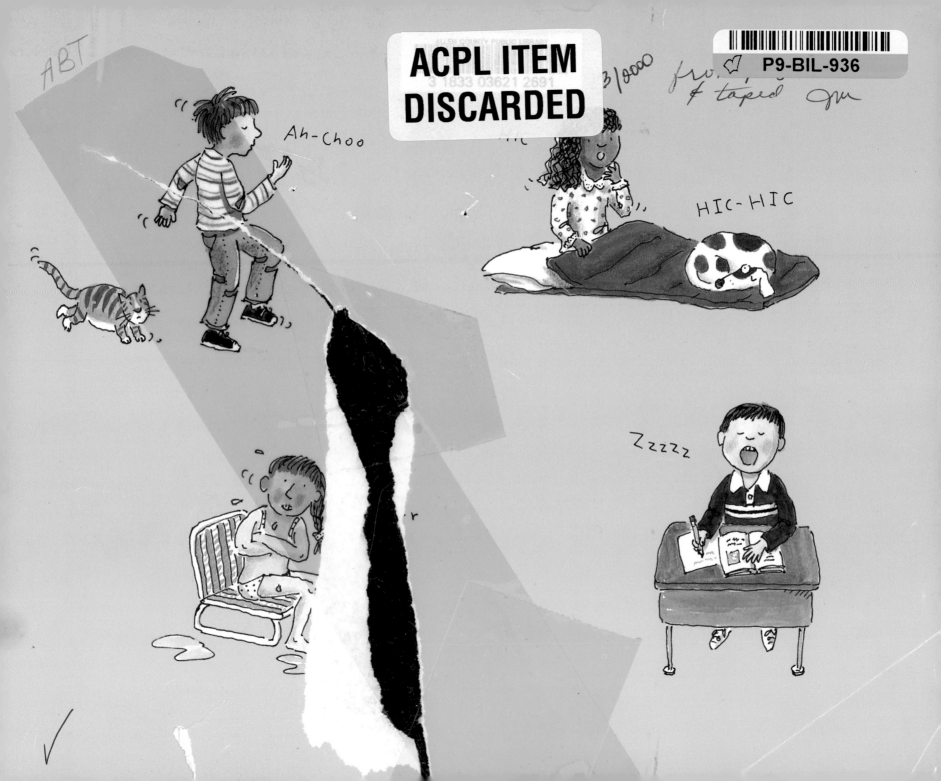

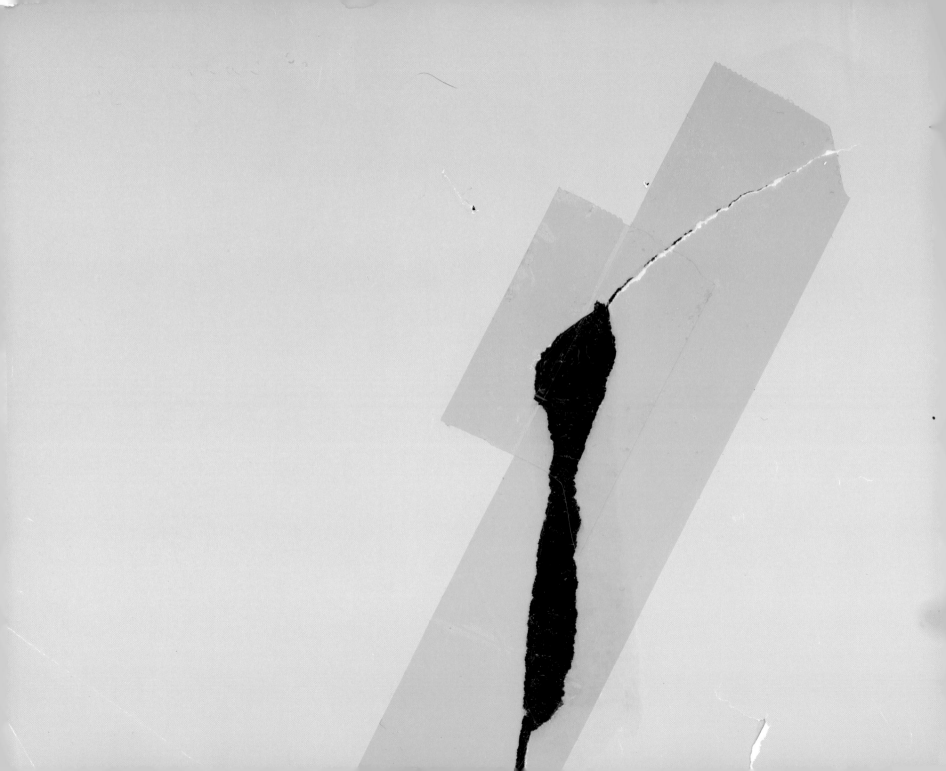

Why I Sneeze, Shiver, Hiccup, and YAWN

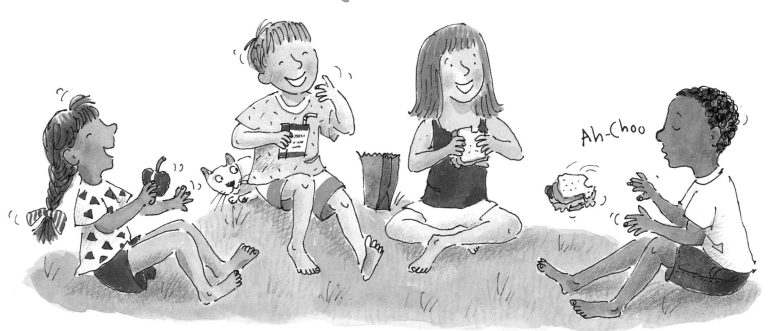

Ah-Choo

by Melvin Berger • illustrated by Paul Meisel

HarperCollins Publishers

The illustrations for this book were created with pen, ink, watercolor, wash and pastel on Arches Lanaquarelle hot-pressed watercolor paper.

Special thanks to Dr. Maurine Packard
of Flushing Hospital for her expert advice.

The *Let's-Read-and-Find-Out Science* book series was originated by Dr. Franklyn M. Branley, Astronomer Emeritus and former Chairman of the American Museum–Hayden Planetarium, and was formerly co-edited by him and Dr. Roma Gans, Professor Emeritus of Childhood Education, Teachers College, Columbia University. Text and illustrations for each of the books in the series are checked for accuracy by an expert in the relevant field. For more information about Let's-Read-and-Find-Out Science books, write to HarperCollins Children's Books, 10 East 53rd Street, New York, NY 10022 or visit our Web site at http://www.harperchildrens.com.

HarperCollins®, ☕®, and Let's Read-and-Find-Out Science® are trademarks of HarperCollins Publishers Inc.

Library of Congress Cataloging-in-Publication Data
Berger, Melvin.
　　Why I sneeze, shiver, hiccup, and yawn / by Melvin Berger ; illustrated by Paul Meisel.
　　　p.　　cm. — (Let's-read-and-find-out science. Stage 2)
　　Rev. ed. of: Why I cough, sneeze, shiver, hiccup, & yawn. New York : Crowell, c1983.
　　Summary: An introduction to reflex acts that explains why we sneeze, shiver, hiccup, and yawn.
　　ISBN 0-06-028144-8. — ISBN 0-06-028143-X (lib. bdg.). — ISBN 0-06-445193-3 (pbk.)
　　I. Reflexes—Juvenile literature. [I. Reflexes.]　I. Meisel, Paul, ill.　II. Berger, Melvin. Why I sneeze, shiver, hiccup, and yawn.
III. Title.　IV. Series.
QP372.B3964　2000
612.7'4—dc21
98-55542
CIP
AC

Typography by Elynn Cohen
1　2　3　4　5　6　7　8　9　10
❖
Newly illustrated edition
Previously published as Why I Cough, Sneeze, Shiver, Hiccup, and Yawn

Why I
Sneeze, Shiver,
HICCUP, and YAWN

Yawn

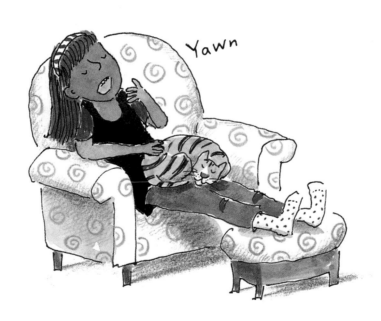

You are playing hide-and-seek. You've found a good hiding place. You want to be as quiet as you can. All of a sudden—KA-CHOO! You sneeze. Everyone knows where you are.

Why do you sneeze—even when you don't want to?

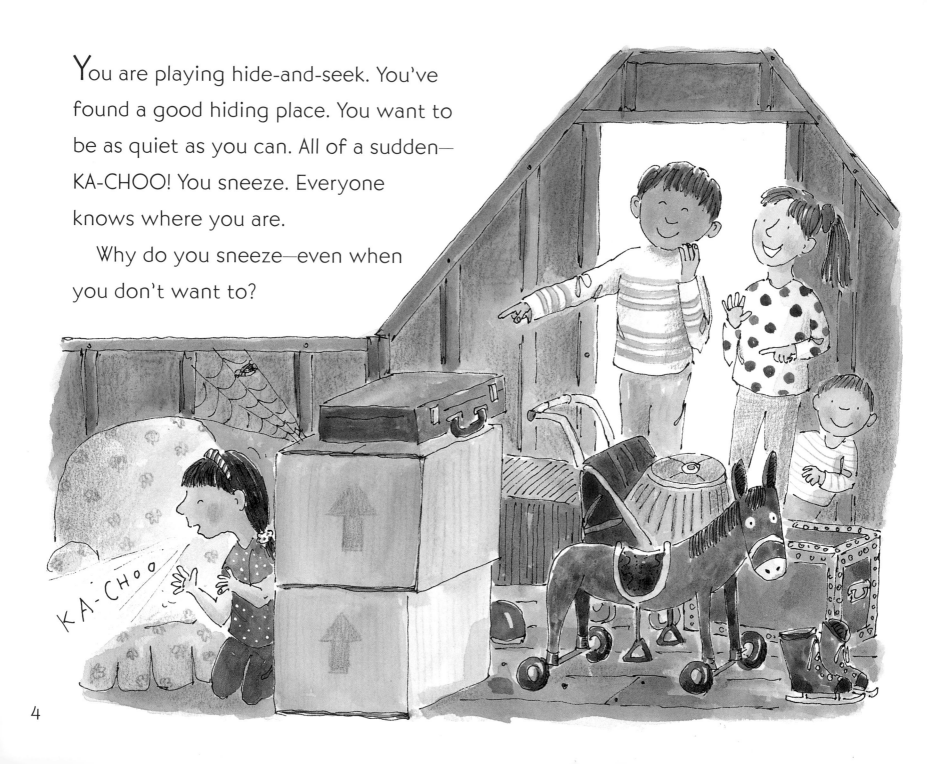

You are eating lunch with your friends. You are in the middle of telling them a story. All at once you hiccup. HIC! Your friends start to laugh. HIC! You try to stop. HIC! But you can't. HIC!

Why do you hiccup—even when you don't want to?

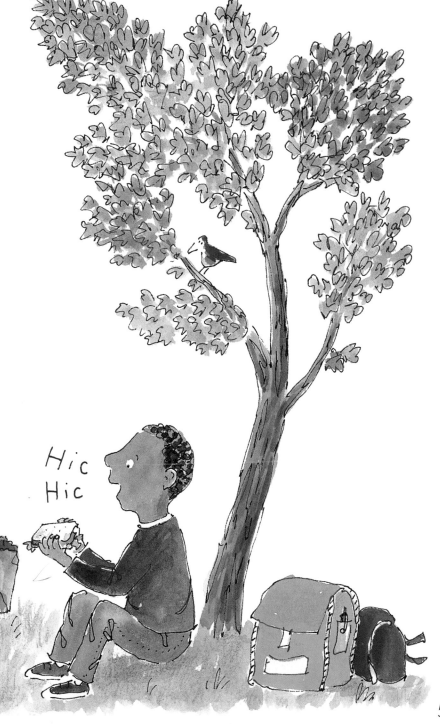

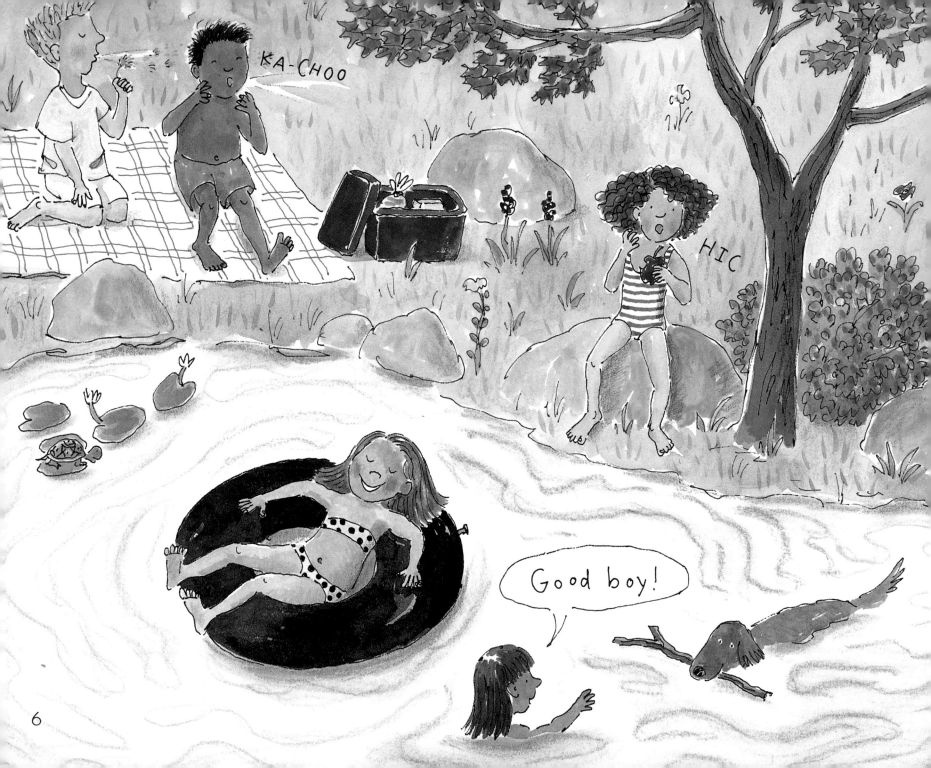

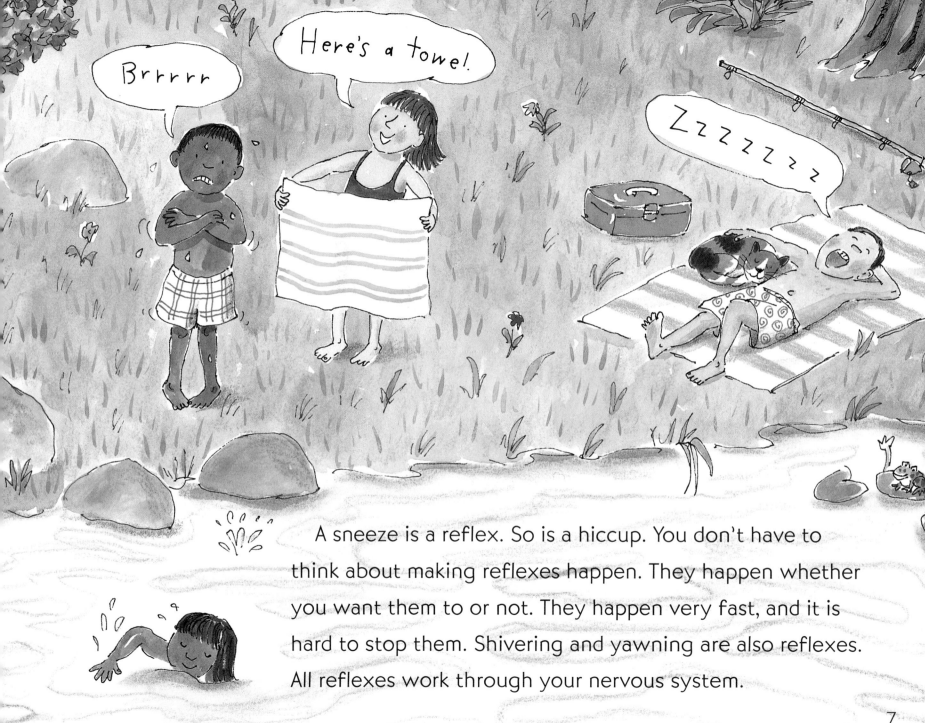

A sneeze is a reflex. So is a hiccup. You don't have to think about making reflexes happen. They happen whether you want them to or not. They happen very fast, and it is hard to stop them. Shivering and yawning are also reflexes. All reflexes work through your nervous system.

7

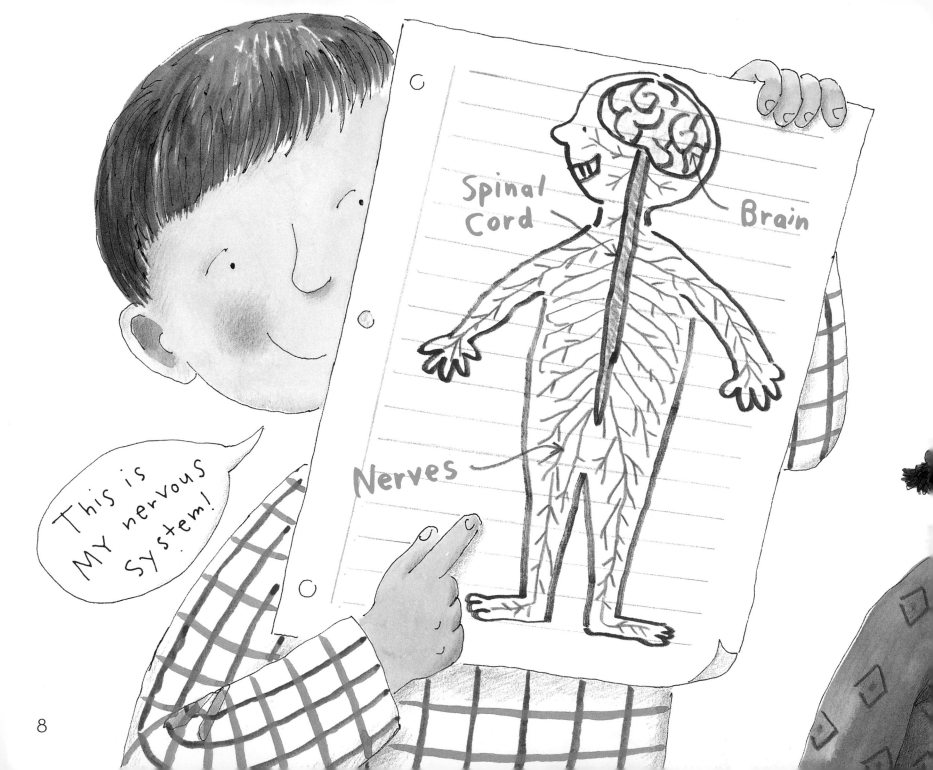

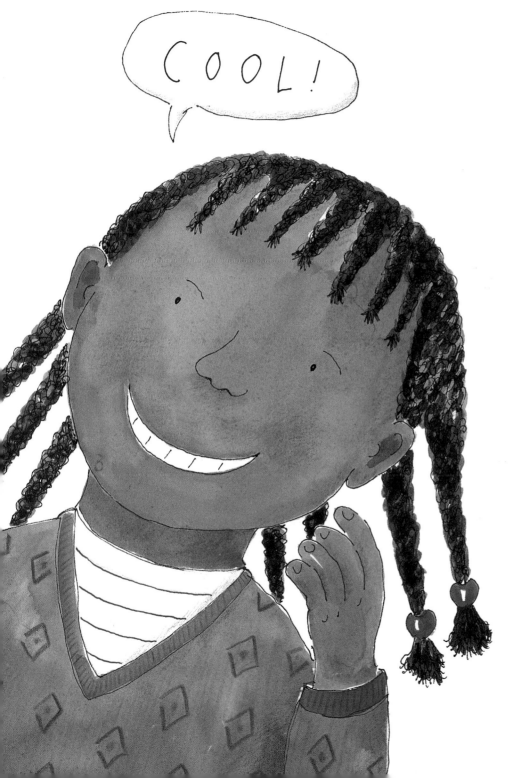

Your nervous system is made up of two parts. One part is the nerves. The nerves look like long, thin threads. They reach all over your body.

The other part is the spinal cord and brain. The spinal cord is a thick bundle of nerves. It is inside your spine, or backbone. The brain is at the upper end of the spinal cord. It is made up of billions of tiny nerves.

Nerves are like telephone wires. They carry messages back and forth. The brain and spinal cord are like the main office of the telephone company. All the messages must go through here.

9

Suppose you put your finger on a hot stove. The nerves in your hand sense that the stove is hot. They send out a message. The message speeds along nerves from your hand to your spinal cord. Here the message passes to a different nerve. This nerve controls the muscles that move your arm.

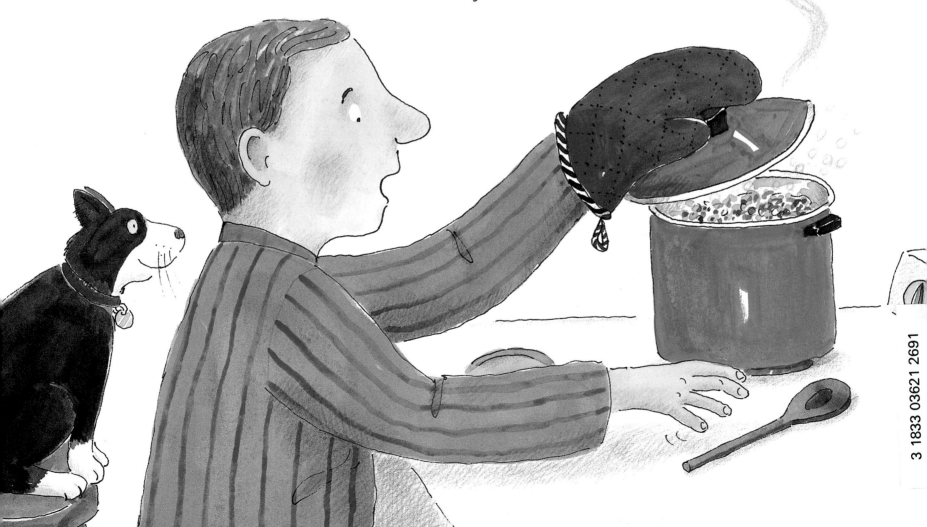

A signal flashes through the nerve. It tells your muscles to move your hand—and fast. Before you even know what hurts, your hand jerks away from the stove.

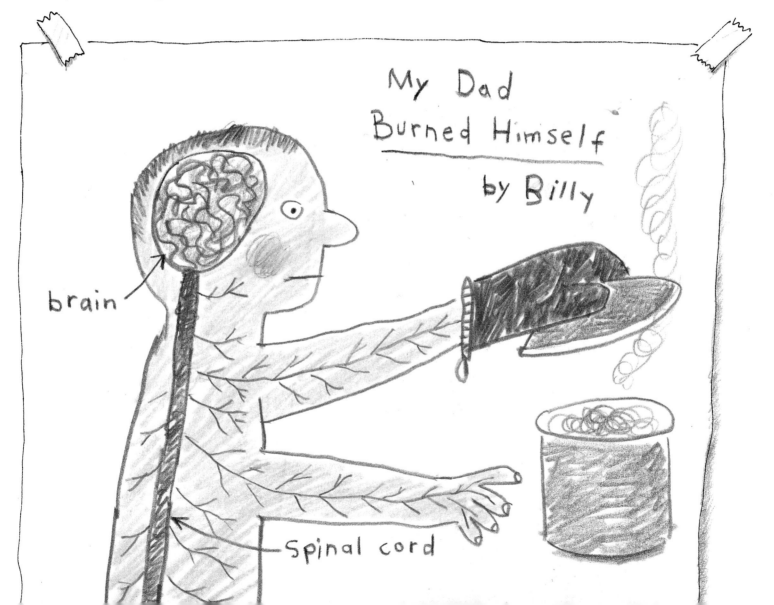

My Dad Burned Himself

by Billy

brain

spinal cord

Pulling your hand off a hot stove is a reflex. It happens very quickly, and it is not completely under your control. It happens automatically, without your having to think about making it happen.

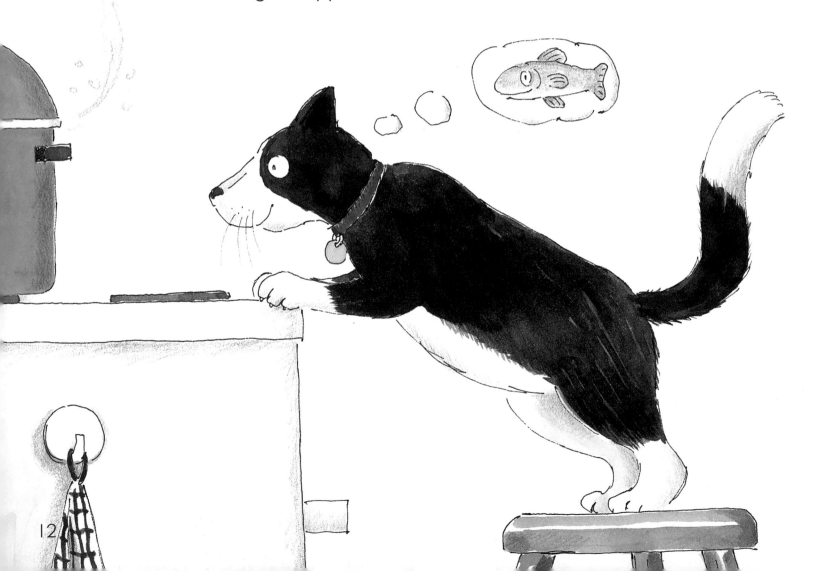

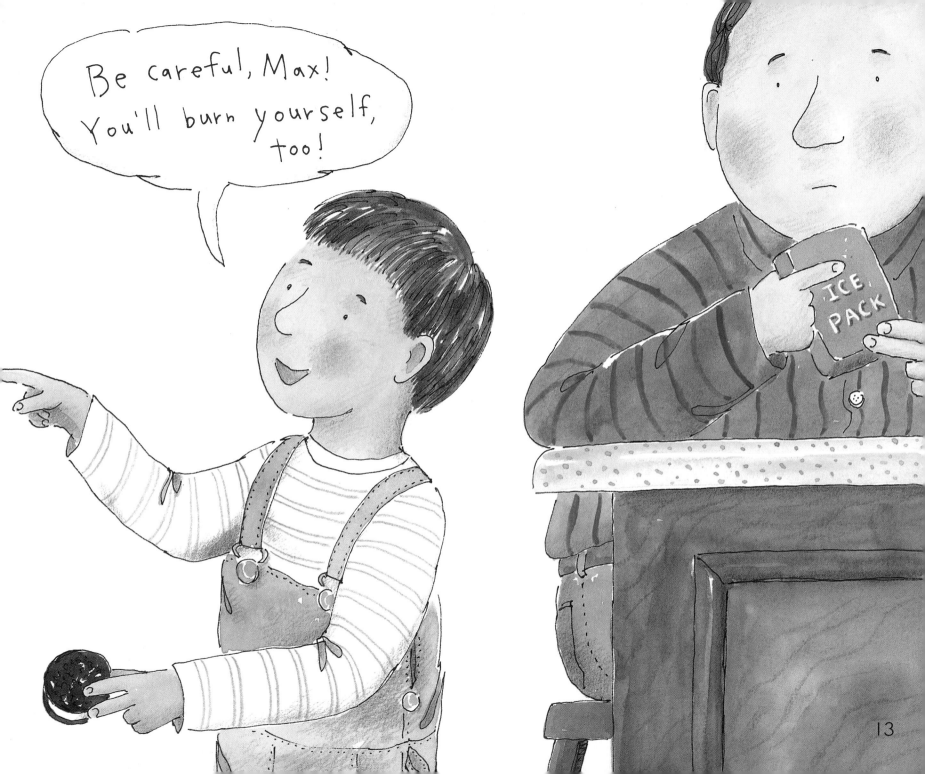

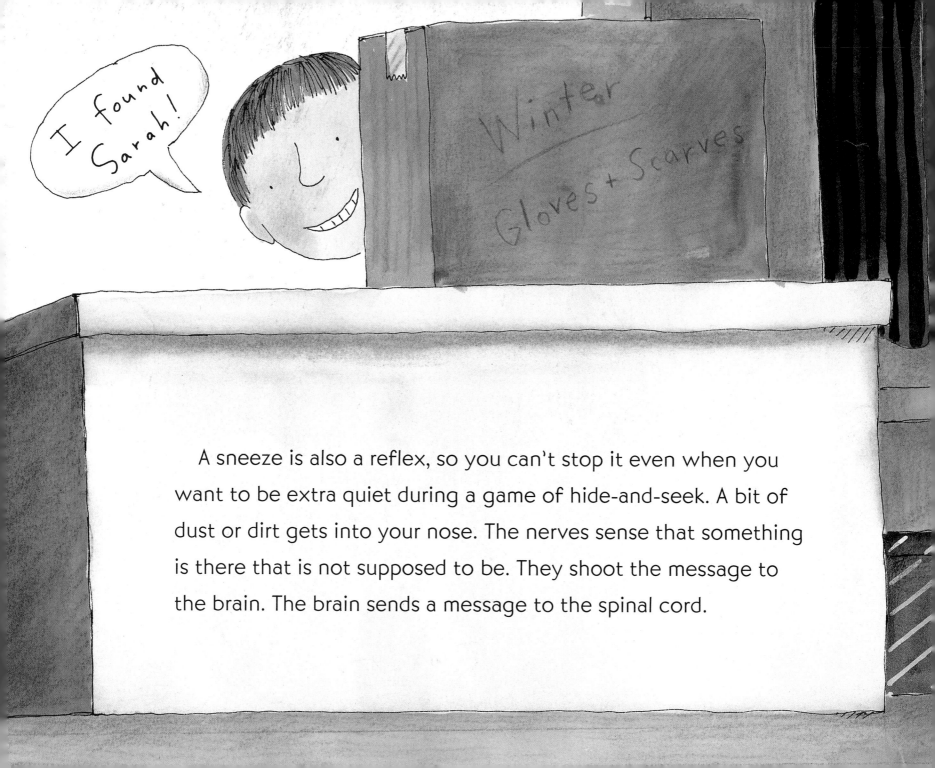

A sneeze is also a reflex, so you can't stop it even when you want to be extra quiet during a game of hide-and-seek. A bit of dust or dirt gets into your nose. The nerves sense that something is there that is not supposed to be. They shoot the message to the brain. The brain sends a message to the spinal cord.

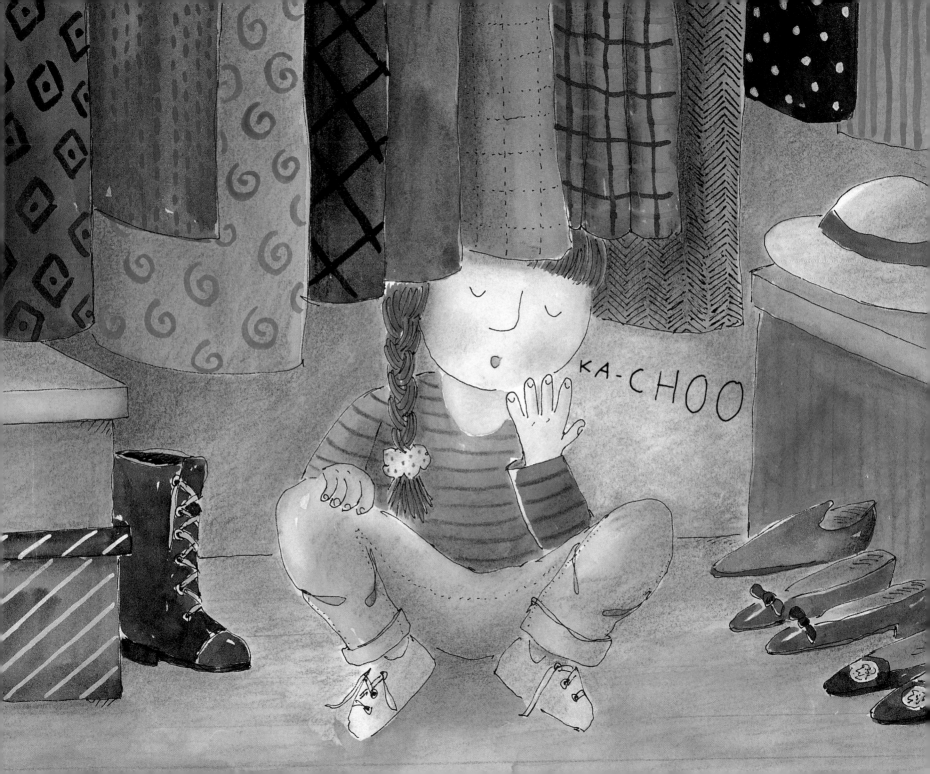

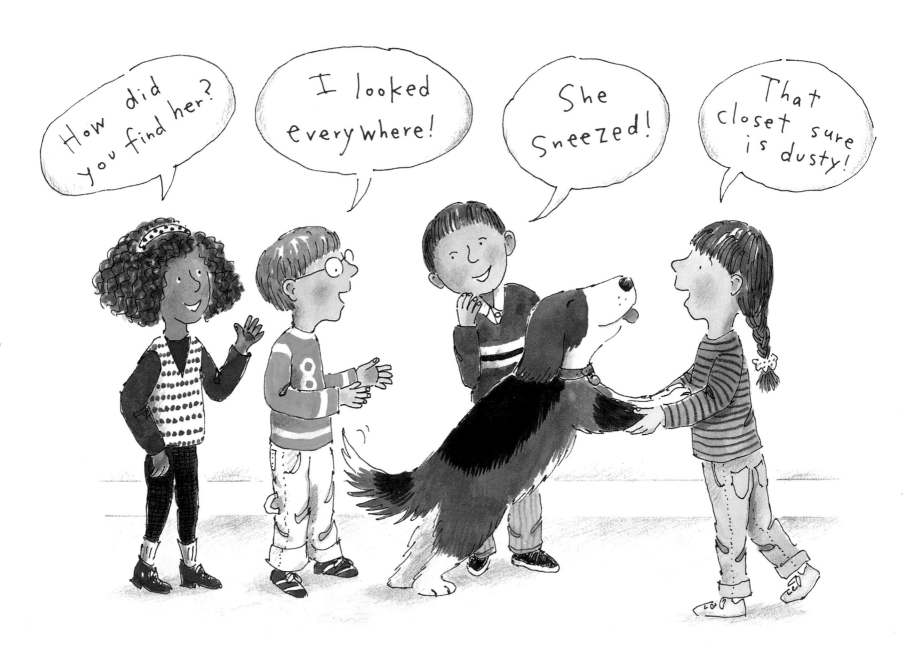

In the spinal cord, the message passes to other nerves that go to your diaphragm and belly muscles. The muscles contract and cause your lungs to send up a blast of air. KA-CHOO! You sneeze. The sneeze blows the dust or dirt out of your nose.

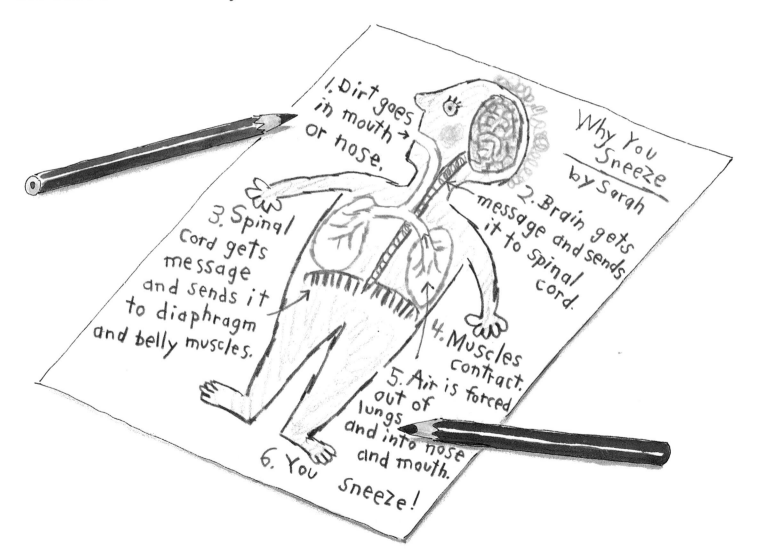

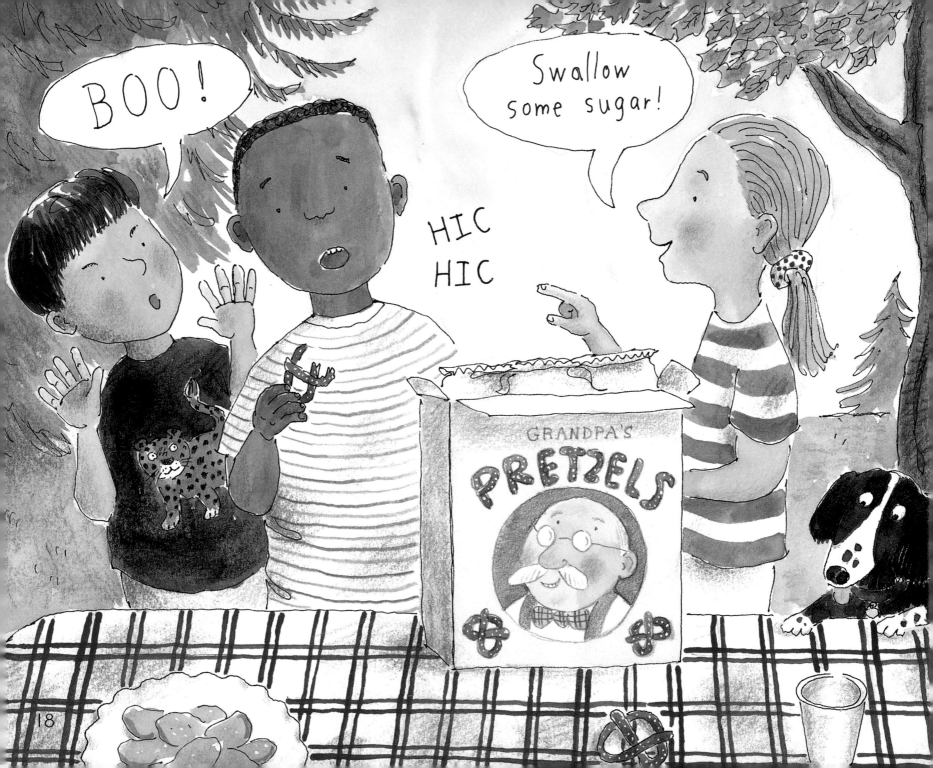

No one knows exactly why hiccups happen. We do know how they work. A message races to your spinal cord. From there a nerve sends out a signal that makes you take in a big gulp of air. But at that moment your throat closes. The air bumps against your closed throat. It makes a sound—HIC! It is a hiccup. The sound gives the hiccup its name.

The hiccup is a reflex. A drink of water may make the hiccups go away.

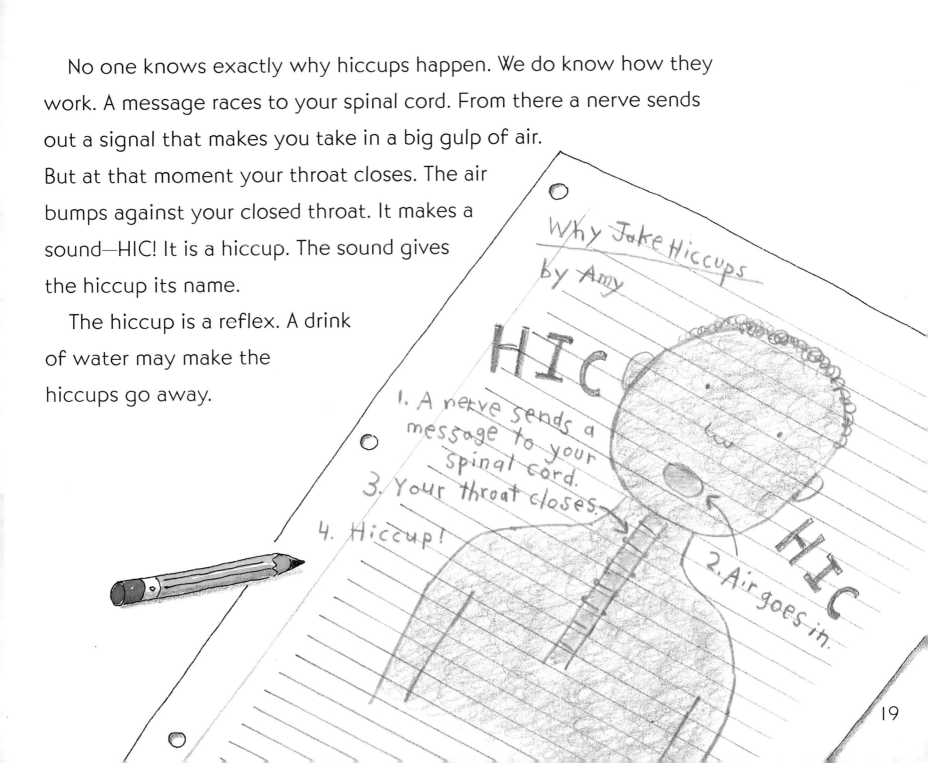

Why Jake Hiccups
by Amy

HIC

1. A nerve sends a message to your spinal cord.
3. Your throat closes.
4. Hiccup!
2. Air goes in.
HIC

A shiver is a reflex just like sneezing and a hiccup. If you step out of a warm bath into a cool room, the nerves in your skin feel that it is cold in the room. They carry the message to nerves in your spinal cord.

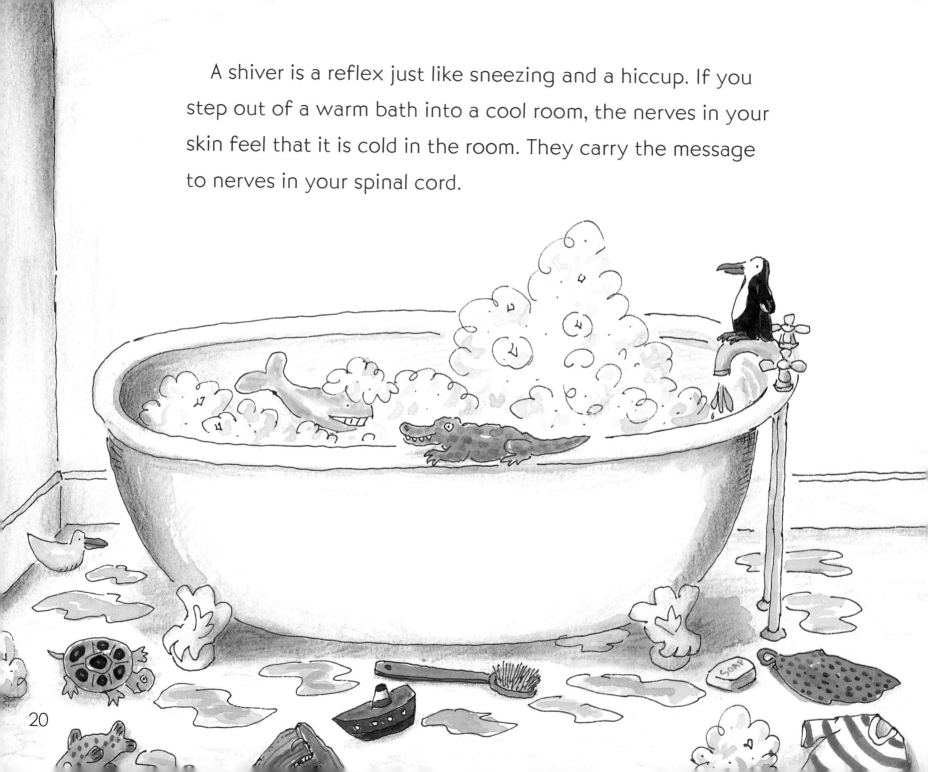

From the spinal cord the message races through other nerves. All over your body, muscles quickly tighten and loosen, tighten and loosen. You are shivering. The moving muscles produce heat. The shivers warm you up.

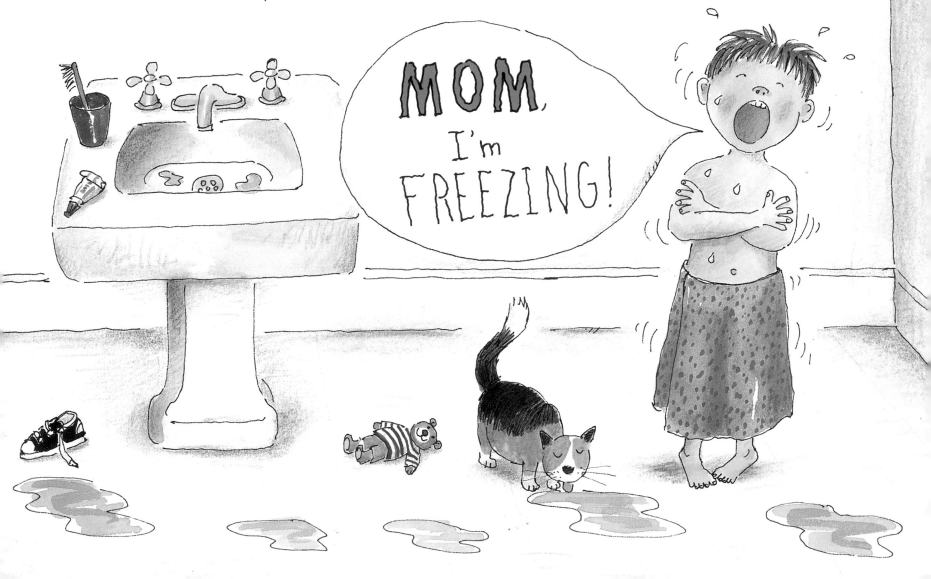

Have you ever tried to hold back a yawn? It is very hard
to do. A yawn is another reflex.

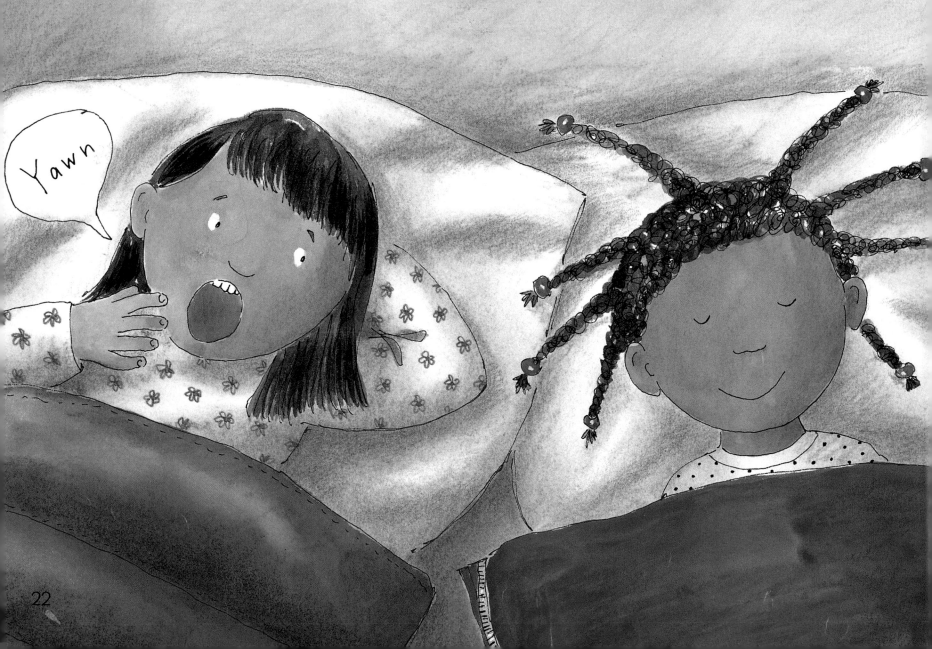

A yawn begins when the lungs have too little oxygen in them. Nerves signal the muscles around your jaw to pull apart. You yawn, and as you do, you take an extra-deep breath of air. With more oxygen in your lungs, you feel a little less sleepy.

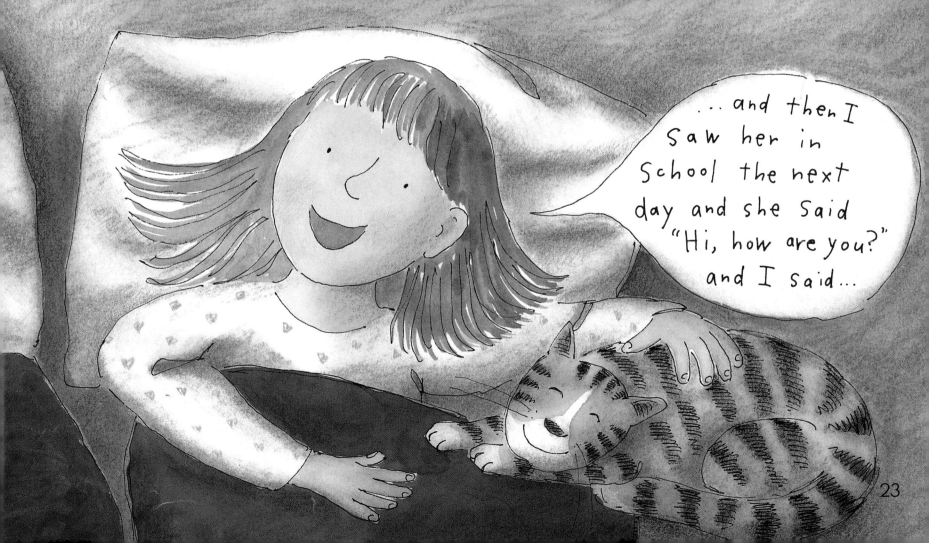

A reflex you can see happens in your eyes. Go into a bright room. After a few minutes, look in a mirror. The black part of your eye—that's the pupil—will be small. Then close your eyes for a few minutes and look in the mirror again.

Your pupils will be big and round.

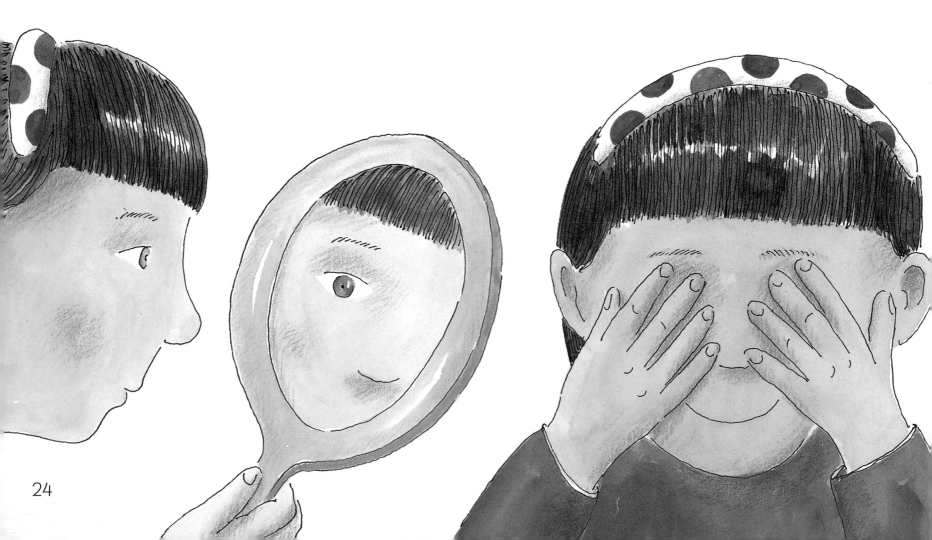

If you wait a few moments with your eyes open in the same room, you will notice that your pupils have gotten small again.

A reflex makes the pupils in your eyes grow larger when there is too little light. This lets more light into your eyes. A reflex also makes your pupils grow smaller in bright light.

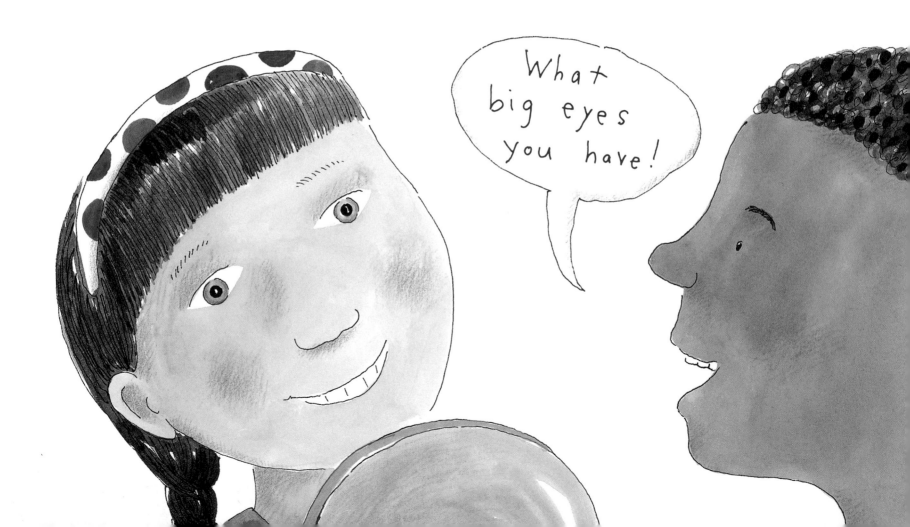

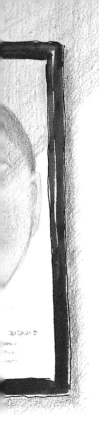

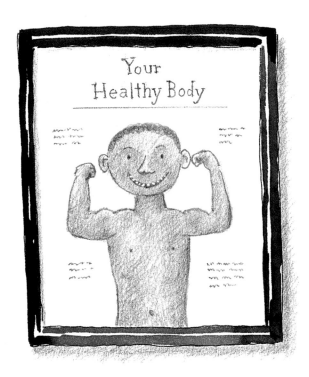

Your Healthy Body

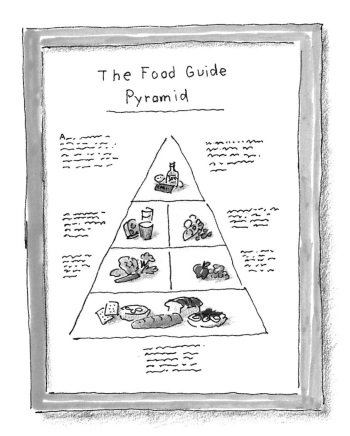

The Food Guide Pyramid

Doctors sometimes test reflexes. Have you ever had the test? You sit on a table with your legs hanging down. The doctor taps just below the knee. The tool that is used looks like a hammer with a rubber head.

Suddenly your leg kicks up. This is a reflex. It is sometimes called the patellar reflex, or knee jerk. A strong patellar reflex is usually a sign of a healthy nervous system.

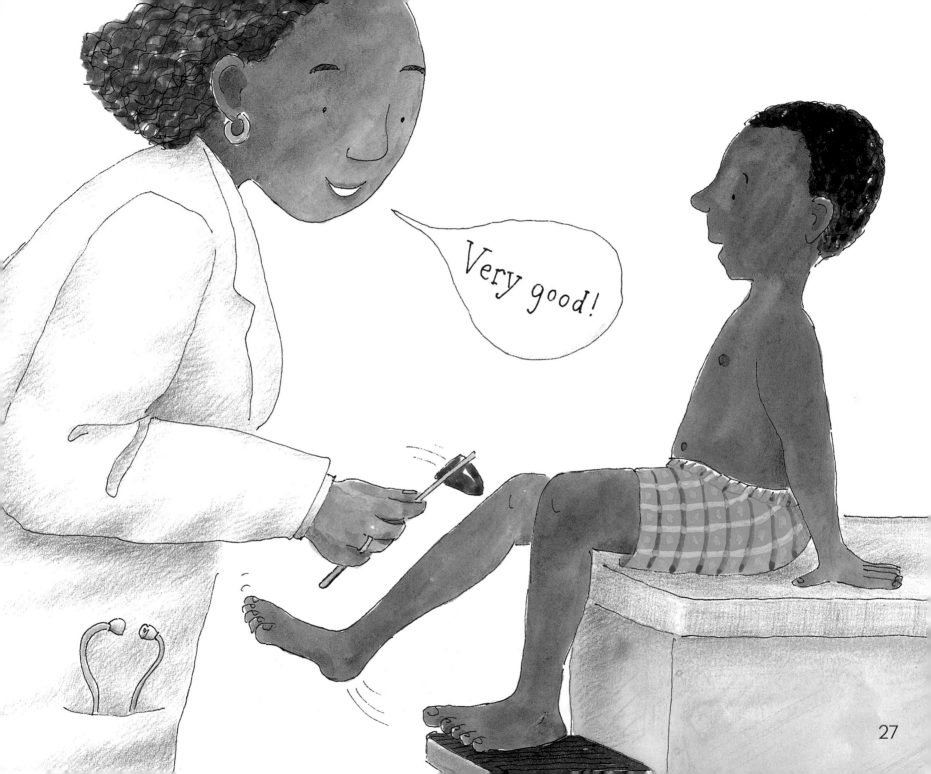

27

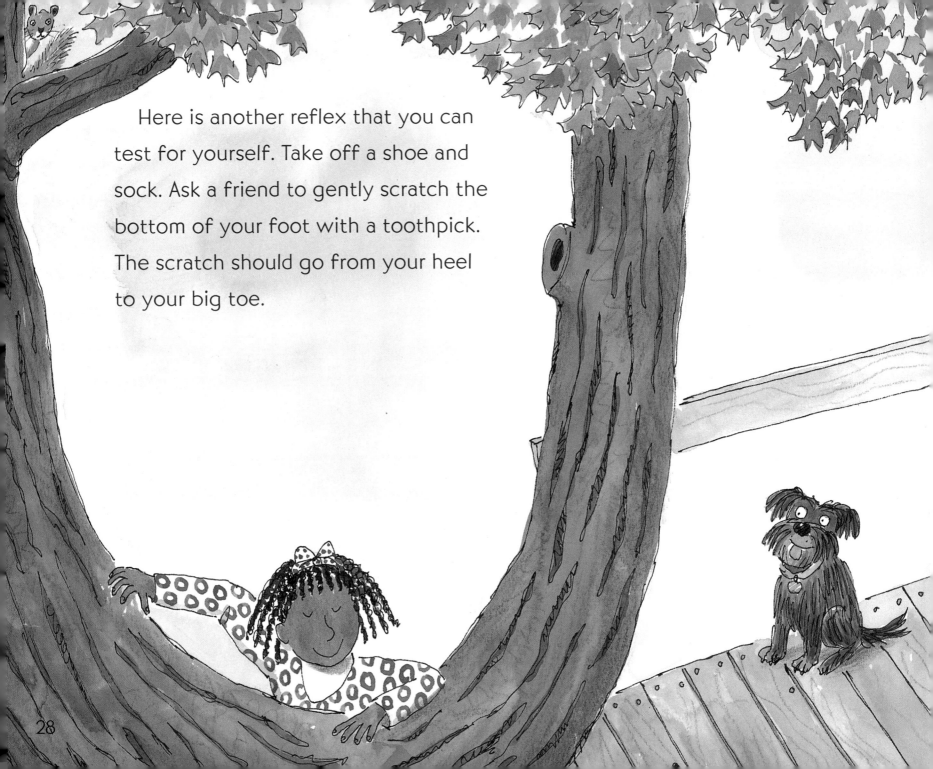

Here is another reflex that you can test for yourself. Take off a shoe and sock. Ask a friend to gently scratch the bottom of your foot with a toothpick. The scratch should go from your heel to your big toe.

Watch your toes slowly bend down. This is called the plantar reflex. It probably helps people walk on rough ground or climb trees barefooted.

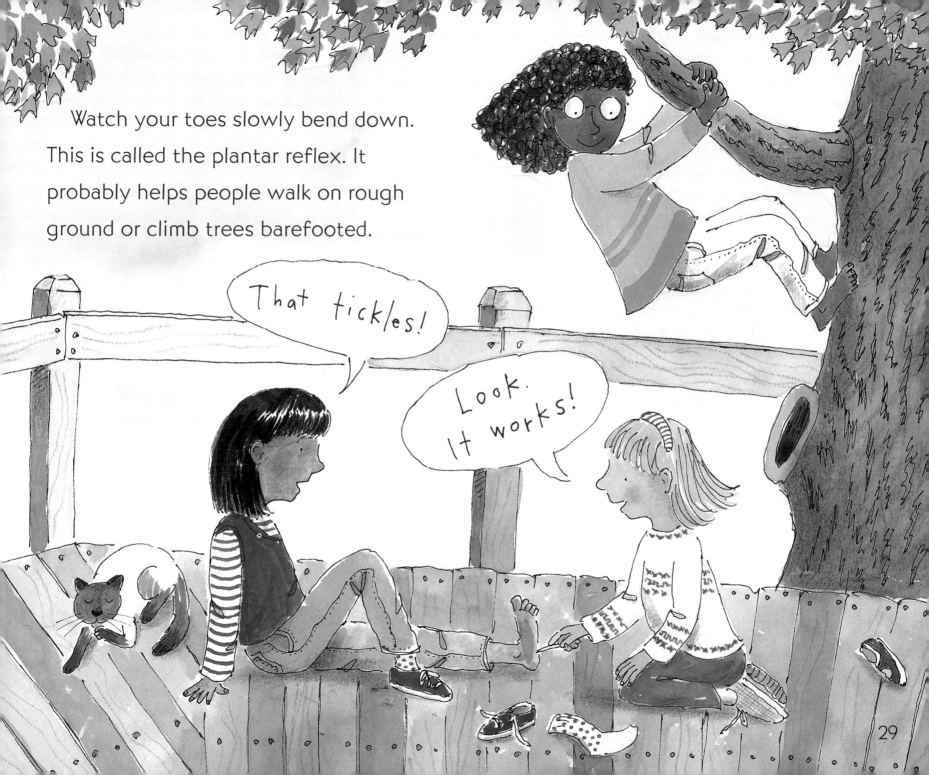

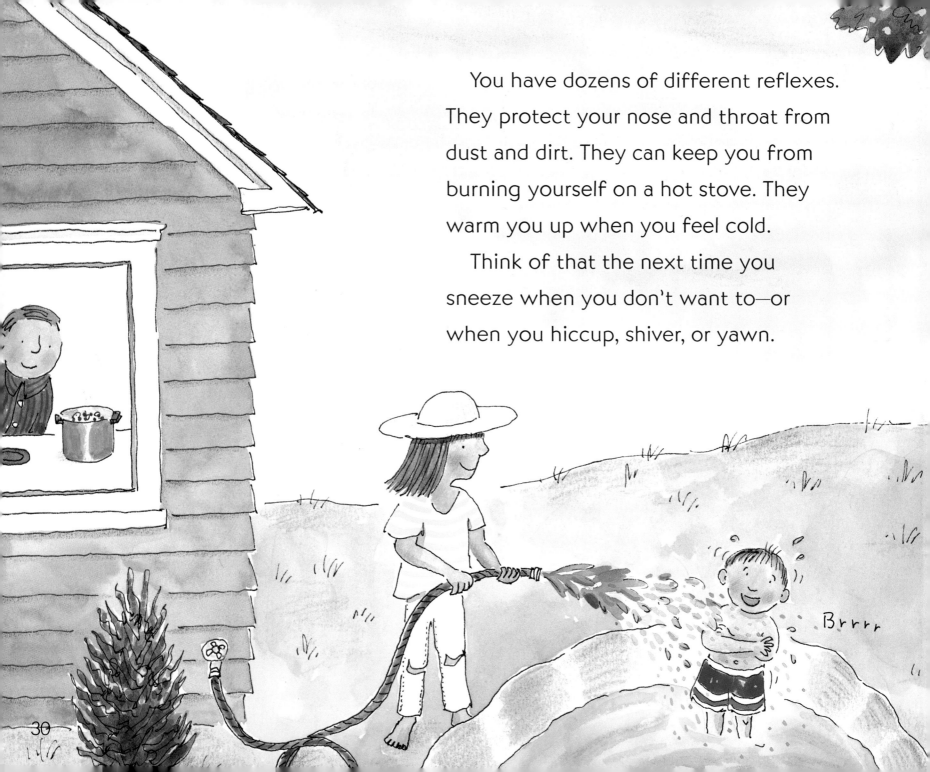

You have dozens of different reflexes. They protect your nose and throat from dust and dirt. They can keep you from burning yourself on a hot stove. They warm you up when you feel cold.

Think of that the next time you sneeze when you don't want to—or when you hiccup, shiver, or yawn.

Brrrr

30

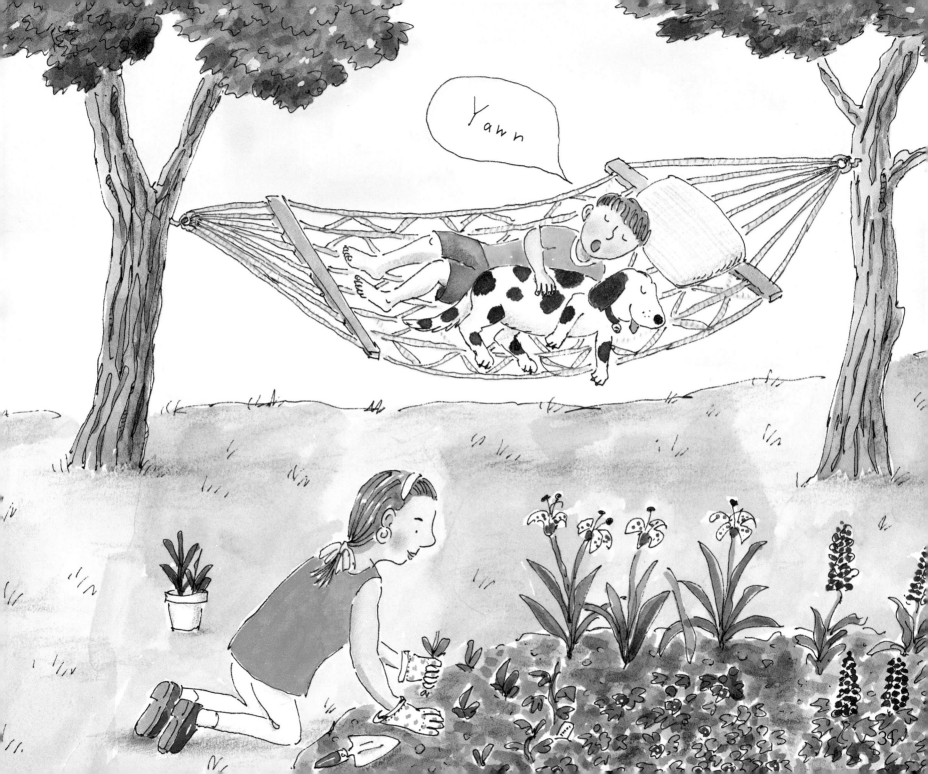

Things to Think About

- What happens to your body when you get cold, besides shivering? You get goose bumps! Goose bumps appear when tiny muscles attached to each hair contract, pulling the hair and skin straight up. The raised hairs are supposed to trap air and body heat close to you, to keep you warm.

- You also get goose bumps when you're scared. Animals do, too. Have you ever seen a cat when it is afraid? When its fur stands up, the cat looks bigger and scarier.

- What happens when you get dust in your eyes? How does this reflex action protect your eyes? Can you think of some other reflex actions?

  - How are reflex actions different from habits like making your bed and brushing your teeth?

  - What are some of the changes that happen in your body when you see or hear something really scary? Does your heart beat faster and your breath get shorter? Do your palms get sweaty? How do you think these things protect and prepare your body for the "fight or flight" reflex?

  - Do you have a baby in the family or neighborhood? What are some reflexes babies have that you don't? The "startle" reflex happens when a baby falls backward a little way and throws out his arms and legs like he wants to grab hold of something. If touched on the cheek, a reflex called the rooting reflex causes a baby's head to turn to find a mother's breast or bottle.

Test Your Reflexes

- See how a loud noise stimulates a friend's blinking reflex. Clap your hands loudly about 6 inches from your friend's face. (Be careful not to get too close!) Your friend will blink right away, as his or her eyelids close automatically to protect his or her eyes. If you do the test many times, can your friend eventually stop the reflex from happening?
- Crush a piece of notebook paper to make a paper ball. Stand on one side of a glass door while a friend stands on the other side. Have your friend throw the paper ball at your face. Does it make you blink? Try hard not to blink your eyes. Can you do it?
- The next time you feel a sneeze coming, try to keep your eyes open until the sneeze has passed. You won't be able to! What function do you think this serves?

Fun Facts

- There are many folk remedies for hiccups. Some of the strangest include covering your head with a wastebasket while a friend taps on it; spitting on a rock and then turning it over; drinking nine swallows of water from your grandfather's cup without taking a breath; and wetting a piece of red thread with your tongue, sticking the string to your forehead, and then looking at it.

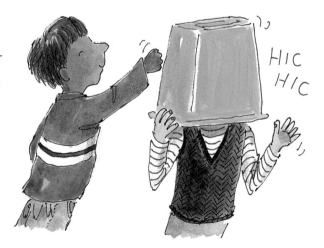

HIC
HIC

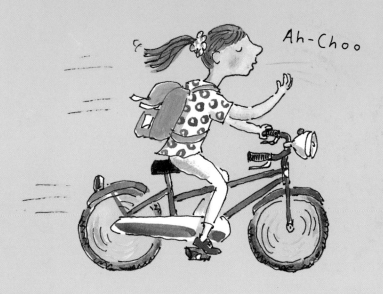

Ah-Choo

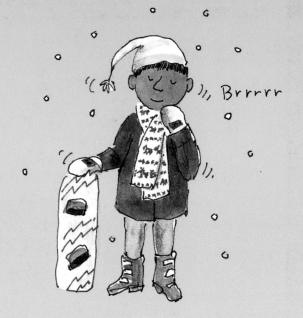

Brrrrr

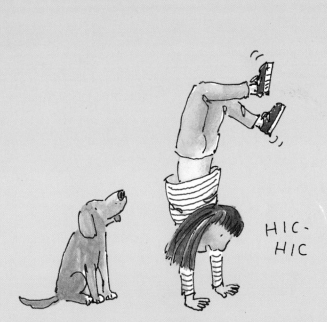

HIC-
HIC

Yawn

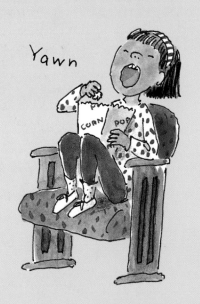